The Ultimate
Keto Chaffle
Recipes Book

An Impeccable Guide
With 50 Mouthwatering
Recipes To Burn Fat And
Boost Your Metabolism.

Vera J. Wren

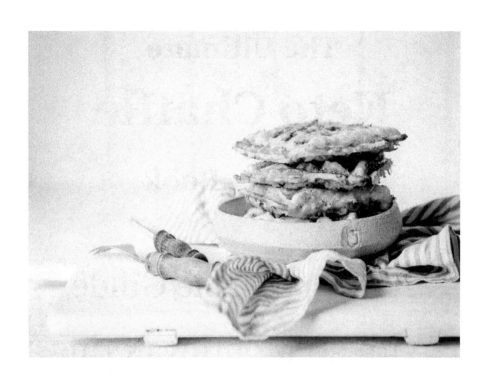

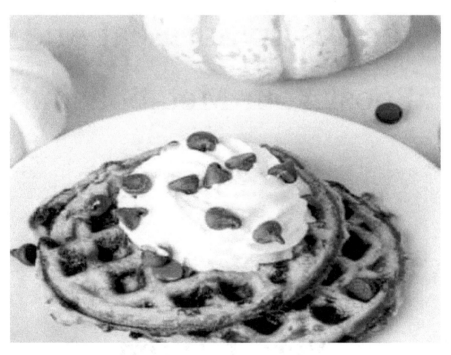

TABLE OF CONTENTS

allowed with the express written consent from the Publisher. All additional right reserved.

The information in the following pages is broadly considered a truthful and accurate account of facts and as such, any inattention, use, or misuse of the information in question by the reader will render any resulting actions solely under their purview. There are no scenarios in which the publisher or the original author of this work can be in any fashion deemed liable for any hardship or damages that may befall them after undertaking information described herein.

Additionally, the information in the following pages is intended only for informational purposes and should thus be thought of as universal. As befitting its nature, it is presented without assurance regarding its prolonged validity or interim quality. Trademarks that are mentioned are done without written consent and can in no way be considered an endorsement from the trademark holder.

INTRODUCTION

Keto Diet is a high-fat, low-carb diet that is an increasingly popular way to lose weight. Keto is short for "ketosis", which occurs when the body has depleted its sugar stores, so it burns stored fat instead of glucose in order to produce energy.

Losing weight on a keto diet sounds pretty easy; just eat a few bacon sandwiches and you'll be slimmer in no time. However, there are drawbacks to this diet, including very low levels of vegetables and fruit (so important for fiber and other nutrients) as well as constipation from lack of dietary fiber. Here are some tips:

- It's important to drink plenty of water, not only because you may be eating more sodium than you need, but because staying hydrated will help your body process proteins and fats more efficiently.

- For best results, stay away from most fruits and vegetables. Some berries are allowed; others aren't. Vegetables that are considered "low in carbs" or "leafy greens" are fine—but there is a difference between low-carb and high-fiber. As a rule of thumb, if it looks like it has the texture of tree bark or is covered with seeds or bulbs (e.g., artichokes), it probably has a lot of carbs and should be avoided.

- Be careful with spices, which tend to have a lot of sugar; salt is OK. It can be easy to go overboard on spices.

- Eat plenty of salmon, tuna and egg whites. Meat—including beef, chicken, pork and lamb—should comprise 20 to 25 percent of your total diet. (Be aware that "lean" meat is often not very lean. Be prepared to trim off most of that fat before cooking.) A little bacon or sausage is fine, too.

- Avoid condiments and sauces, including barbecue sauce and ketchup. These are full of sugar and other unhealthy ingredients.

- Drink mostly water (or unsweetened drinks such as tea or coffee). Try to avoid drinks with a lot of added sugar, like fruit juice or alcohol. If you choose to drink wine, go for the dry stuff—red wine is best.

Now, for Chaffles.

What is Chaffle?

Keto chaffle recipe is a versatile and easy-to-make low carb pancake that only requires 2 ingredients. It's a way to satisfy your sweet cravings while staying keto!

Chaffle is made from cheese and eggs. You will need grated cheddar cheese (use any kind of cheese you have on hand) and eggs, beaten together, then fried in a pan with butter or coconut oil.

Chaffles are perfect for a low carb breakfast, lunch or dinner and can be a treat right out of the pan, with butter!

Why Keto and Chaffle is a perfect combination?

Keto Chaffle is a great way to satisfy your sweet cravings while staying 100% in ketosis. It helps you feel fuller for longer but at the same time it's not a high carb treat.

Chaffle gives you a lot of energy and it's an easy way to prepare breakfast if you want it to be ready quickly when you get up or even if you're in a hurry so it can be prepared on the go without any issues.

Keto Chaffle tastes amazing plain, with butter or with any toppings you like and it can also be used as sandwich bread substitute.

KETOGENIC DIET AND ITS BENEFITS

What is Ketogenic Diet?

The ketogenic diet is a low-carb, high-fat diet. This means that the macronutrient ratio of your diet should consist mainly of fat and protein with only a small percentage of carbohydrates.

The idea behind the ketogenic diet is to force your body to use fat rather than glucose as its primary fuel source. When we are in ketosis, we can function on almost any fuel source.

Benefits of the Ketogenic Diet

The benefits of the ketogenic diet are as follows:

1. No need to count calories.

On this diet, you can eat as much as you want. Since there are no grains, the carbohydrates in the diet are very low, and so you will not take in many calories.

2. There is no need to spend a lot of money on expensive foods.

Since this diet is high in fat, one of the cheapest sources of fat is chicken thighs and legs and other skinless poultry parts or meats from around the animal, such as organ meats (heart, liver, etc.).

3. Low levels of Beta-hydroxybutyrate (ketone body) is suitable for brain health

The ketogenic diet can increase the level of ketone bodies by 10 times than normal dietary levels through fat metabolism.

4. Decreased risk of heart disease

Many people can lower their LDL (bad) cholesterol by 75-90% and triglyceride levels by 60%.

5. Less inflammation

Because there are no carbohydrates in the ketogenic diet, your body becomes very efficient at burning ketones as fuel. This is excellent news if you have an autoimmune disorder like rheumatoid arthritis or Crohn's disease because inflammation is often linked to autoimmune problems.

6. Fast weight loss

People usually start losing weight within two weeks of starting the diet.

7. Increased energy levels

The ketogenic diet can increase your energy levels because you will be consuming a high-fat diet with very few carbohydrates.

8. No constant hunger

When people are on a ketogenic diet, they are in "ketosis." This means that their bodies are using fat as an almost complete fuel source. This is the opposite of how most people function in a non-ketogenic state, which usually involves using carbohydrates (sugars) as a practically whole fuel source. Because the ketogenic diet is so different, the body is forced to use fat as its primary fuel source to function. This means you won't be hungry all the time once you get the hang of it.

9. No need for cheat meals

Since carbohydrates are reduced in this diet, cheating on the ketogenic diet will not help you lose weight because your body does not have carbohydrates stored to keep your metabolism running, being that fat is used instead of sugar/carbs.

10. No need to buy expensive supplements

Since the diet is not very restrictive, you won't need to buy many supplements besides vitamin D3 if you are deficient.

11. You can gain muscle and lose fat at the same time

When you do strength training with a ketogenic diet, the weight loss is due to body fat (adipose tissue), not muscle mass. Many people find it difficult to lose weight because they are losing muscle mass and body fat, which is not suitable for overall health. However, because this diet encourages protein consumption at every meal, as well as healthy fats, your amino acid intake will be sufficient to preserve your muscles without inhibiting your weight loss.

Foods Allowed

Here is the list of foods you can eat during the ketogenic diet:

1. Meat, poultry, fish, shellfish, and eggs from pasture-fed animals (animals are fed a grass-fed diet)
2. Fish and seafood caught in the wild
3. Eggs from pastured hens
4. Vegetables, including root vegetables such as beets and carrots and leafy greens such as spinach and kale.

5. Healthy fats such as coconut oil or olive oil that can be used in place of butter or other oils (11 grams per day maximum)

6. Nuts and seeds such as macadamia nuts, walnuts, and pumpkin seeds

7. Low to moderate amounts of dairy products such as yogurt and cheese

8. Non-starchy vegetables such as broccoli, cauliflower, and other cruciferous vegetables

9. Fruits

Foods That Are Not Allowed

Foods that are not allowed

When following the keto diet, you will want to avoid eating the following foods:

1. Grains including wheat, oats, rice, and corn

2. Sugar, including honey, maple syrup, and sugar in all its forms

3. Vegetable oils such as canola, sunflower, and soybean oil

4. Trans fats such as margarine and vegetable shortening

5. Juices and sugary drinks such as soda, fruit juices with added sugar or artificial sweeteners, or milk alternatives made with grains such as almond milk

6. Grain-based dairy products such as butter and yogurt

7. Legumes such as beans, soybeans, and peanuts

8. Starchy vegetables such as potatoes, peas, and corn

9. Processed foods of any kind, including sauces and any food that contains a high percentage of preservatives

10. Beer (pure alcohol)

11. Low-fat or nonfat dairy products such as yogurt and cheese (dairy products that are low in fat but have carbohydrates)

12. Fruit juices with added sugars or artificial sweeteners

Volume (liquid)

US Customary	Metric
1/8 teaspoon	.6 ml
1/4 teaspoon	1.2 ml
1/2 teaspoon	2.5 ml
3/4 teaspoon	3.7 ml
1 teaspoon	5 ml
1 tablespoon	15 ml
2 tablespoon or 1 fluid ounce	30 ml
1/4 cup or 2 fluid ounces	59 ml
1/3 cup	79 ml
1/2 cup	118 ml
2/3 cup	158 ml
3/4 cup	177 ml
1 cup or 8 fluid ounces	237 ml
2 cups or 1 pint	473 ml
4 cups or 1 quart	946 ml
8 cups or 1/2 gallon	1.9 liters
1 gallon	3.8 liters

Weight (mass)

US contemporary (ounces)	Metric (grams)
1/2 ounce	14 grams
1 ounce	28 grams
3 ounces	85 grams
3.53 ounces	100 grams
4 ounces	113 grams
8 ounces	227 grams
12 ounces	340 grams
16 ounces or 1 pound	454 grams

Volume Equivalents (liquid)*

3 teaspoons	1 tablespoon	0.5 fluid ounce
2 tablespoons	1/8 cup	1 fluid ounce
4 tablespoons	1/4 cup	2 fluid ounces
5 1/3 tablespoons	1/3 cup	2.7 fluid ounces
8 tablespoons	1/2 cup	4 fluid ounces
12 tablespoons	3/4 cup	6 fluid ounces
16 tablespoons	1 cup	8 fluid ounces
2 cups	1 pint	16 fluid ounces

BREAKFAST RECIPES

1. Chicken Cauli Chaffle

Preparation Time: 27 minutes

Cooking Time: 12 minutes

Servings: 2

Ingredients:

- Chicken: 3-4 pieces or ½ cup when done
- Garlic: 2 cloves (finely grated)
- Egg: 2
- Salt: As per your taste
- Green onion: 1 stalk
- Soy Sauce: 1 tablespoon
- Cauliflower Rice: 1 cup
- Mozzarella cheese: 1 cup
- Black pepper: ¼ teaspoon or as per your taste
- White pepper: ¼ teaspoon or as per your taste

Directions:

1. Melt some butter in an oven and set aside, then cook the chicken in a skillet using salt and a cup of water to boil. With the lid closed, cook for 18 minutes. Once done, put off the heat and shred the chicken into pieces, then discard all bones.

2. Using another mixing bowl prepare a mix containing peppers (white and black), soy sauce, cauliflower rice, grated garlic, beaten egg with the shredded chicken pieces. Mix evenly. Preheat and grease the waffle maker. Pour 1/8 cup of mozzarella into the waffle maker with the mixture on the cheese, add another cup (1/8) of mozzarella on the chaffle. With a closed lid, heat the waffle for 5 minutes to a crunch and then remove the chaffle. Repeat for the remaining chaffles mixture to make more batter. Serve by garnishing the chaffle with chopped green onions and enjoy.

Nutrition:
- Calories: 144 kcal
- Cholesterol: 111 mg
- Carbohydrates: 4.7 g
- Protein: 4.7 g
- Fat: 10.2 g

2. Garlic Chicken Chaffle

Preparation Time: 27 minutes

Cooking Time: 12 minutes

Servings: 2

Ingredients:

- Chicken: 3-4 pieces
- Garlic: 1 clove
- Egg: 1
- Salt
- Lemon juice: ½ tablespoon
- Kewpie mayo: 2 tablespoons
- Mozzarella cheese: ½ cup

Directions:

1. Cook the chicken in a skillet using salt and a cup of water to boil. With the lid closed, cook for 18 minutes. Once done, put off the heat and shred the chicken into pieces, then discard all bones. Using another mixing bowl prepare a mix containing 1/8 cup of cheese, Kewpie mayo, lemon juice and grated garlic. Mix evenly. Preheat and grease the waffle maker. Arrange chaffles on a baking tray with the chicken, then sprinkle cheese on the chaffles. With a closed lid, heat the waffle for 5 minutes until cheese melts and then remove the chaffle. Repeat

for the remaining chaffles mixture to make more batter. Serve and warm.

Nutrition:
- Calories: 144 kcal
- Cholesterol: 111 mg
- Carbohydrates: 4.7 g
- Protein: 4.7 g

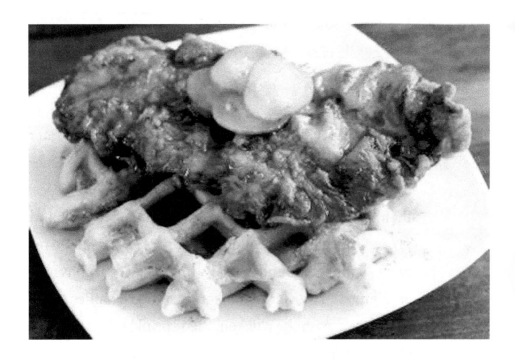

3. Chicken Mozzarella Chaffle

Preparation Time: 12 minutes

Cooking Time: 6 minutes

Servings: 2

Ingredients:

- Chicken: 1 cup
- Mozzarella cheese: 1 cup and 4 tablespoons
- Basil: ½ teaspoon
- Butter: 1 teaspoon
- Egg: 2
- Tomato sauce: 6 tablespoons
- Garlic: ½ tablespoon

Directions:

1. Melt some butter in a pan with shredded chicken added into it and stir for few minutes. Add basil with garlic and set aside. Using a mixing bowl, prepare a mixture containing eggs with cooked chicken and mozzarella cheese, then mix evenly. Preheat and grease a waffle maker. Spread the mixture on the base of the mini-waffle maker evenly, then heat for 5 minutes to a crispy form. Repeat the process for the remaining batter. On a baking tray, arrange the chaffles with tomato sauce and grated cheese to garnish the top. Heat the oven at 399F to melt cheese then serve best hot.

Nutrition:

- Calories: 220 kcal
- Cholesterol: 120 mg
- Carbohydrates: 4.7 g
- Protein: 4.7 g

4. Chicken BBQ Chaffle

Preparation Time: 32 minutes

Cooking Time: 11 minutes

Servings: 2

Ingredients:

- Chicken: 1/2 cup
- BBQ sauce: 1 tablespoon (sugar-free)
- Egg: 1
- Almond flour: 2 tablespoons
- Cheddar cheese: ½ cup
- Butter: 1 tablespoon

Directions:

1. Melt some butter in a pan with shredded chicken added into it and stir for 11 minutes. Using a mixing bowl, prepare a mixture containing all ingredients with the cooked chicken, then mix evenly. Preheat and grease a waffle maker. Spread the mixture on the base of the waffle maker evenly, and then heat for 7 minutes to a crispy form. Repeat the process for the remaining batter. Serve best hot.

Nutrition:

- Calories: 150 kcal
- Cholesterol: 160 mg
- Carbohydrates: 6.4 g
- Protein: 4.7 g

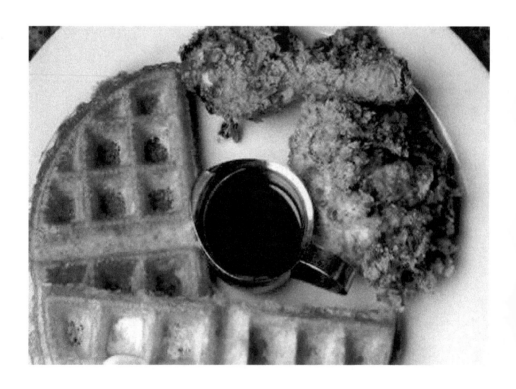

5. Chicken Spinach Chaffle

Preparation Time: 41 minutes

Cooking Time: 11 minutes

Servings: 2

Ingredients:

- Spinach: ½ cup
- Pepper: As per your taste
- Basil: 1 teaspoon
- Chicken: ½ cup boneless
- Shredded mozzarella: half cup
- Garlic powder: 1 tablespoon
- Salt: As per your taste
- Egg: 1
- Onion powder: 1 tablespoon

Directions:

1. Heat the chicken in water to boil, then shred it into pieces and keep aside. Heat the spinach for 9 minutes to strain. Using a mixing bowl, prepare a mixture containing all ingredients with the cooked chicken, then mix evenly. Preheat and grease a waffle maker. Spread the mixture on the base of the waffle maker evenly, and then heat for 7 minutes to a crispy form. Repeat the process for the remaining batter. Serve best crispy with your desired keto sauce.

Nutrition:

- Calories: 200 kcal
- Cholesterol: 98 mg
- Carbohydrates: 3.7 g
- Protein: 4.7 g

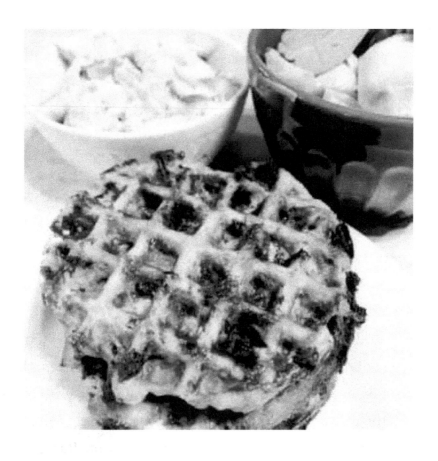

6. Chicken Parmesan Chaffle

Preparation Time: 30 mins

Cooking Time: 5 mins

Servings: 2

Ingredients

- 1/2 Cup Canned Chicken Breast or Leftover Shredded Chicken
- 1/4 Cup Cheddar Cheese
- 1/8 Cup Parmesan Cheese
- 1 Egg
- 1 Teaspoon Italian Seasoning
- 1/8 Teaspoon Garlic Powder
- 1 Teaspoon Cream Cheese, Room Temperature
- Topping Ingredients
- 2 Slices of Provolone Cheese
- 1 Tablespoon Sugar-Free Pizza Sauce I Like Using Rao's Sauces!

Directions:

1. Preheat the mini waffle maker.
2. In a medium-size bowl, add all the ingredients and mix until it's fully incorporated.
3. Add a teaspoon of shredded cheese to the waffle iron for 30 seconds before adding the mixture.

4. This will create the best crust and make it easier to take this heavy chaffle out of the waffle maker when it's done.

5. Pour half of the mixture in the mini waffle maker and cook it for a minimum of 4 to 5 minutes.

6. Repeat the above steps to cook the second Chicken Parmesan Chaffle.

7. Top with a sugar-free pizza sauce and one slice of provolone cheese. I like to sprinkle the top with even more Italian Seasoning too!

Nutrition:

- Calories: 194 kcal
- Cholesterol: 136 mg
- Carbohydrates: 5.9 g
- Protein: 4.7 g

7. Corndog Chaffle

Preparation Time: 45 mins

Cooking Time: 5 mins

Servings: 2

Ingredients

- 2 Eggs
- 1 Cup Mexican Cheese Blend
- 1 Tablespoon Almond Flour
- 1/2 Teaspoon Cornbread Extract
- 1/4 Teaspoon Salt
- Hot Dogs with Hot Dog Sticks
- Optional: For Extra Added Spice Be Sure to Add Diced Jalapenos to This Recipe!

Directions:

1. Preheat corndog waffle maker.
2. In a small bowl, whip the eggs.
3. Add the remaining ingredients, except for the hotdogs
4. Spray the corndog waffle maker with non-stick cooking spray.
5. Fill the corndog waffle maker with the batter halfway filled. (if you want a crispy corndog, add a small amount of cheese 30 seconds before adding the batter)
6. Place a stick in the hot dog.
7. Place the hot dog in the batter and slightly press down.

8. Spread a small amount of batter on top of the hot dog, just enough to fill it.

9. Makes about 4 to 5 chaffle corndogs

10. Cook the corndog chaffles for about 4 minutes or until golden brown.

11. When done, they will easily remove from the corndog waffle maker with a pair of tongs.

12. Serve with mustard, mayo, or sugar-free ketchup!

Nutrition:

- Calories: 200 kcal
- Cholesterol: 120 mg
- Carbohydrates: 4.7 g
- Protein: 4.7 g

8. Burger Bun Chaffle

Preparation Time: 3 mins

Cooking Time: 5 mins

Servings: 2

Ingredients

- 1 Large Egg, Beaten
- 1/2 Cup Shredded Mozzarella
- 1 Tb Almond Flour
- 1/4 Tsp Baking Powder
- 1 Teaspoon Sesame Seeds
- 1 Pinch of Onion Powder

Directions

1. Combine all ingredients
2. Pour half into a mini waffle maker (or split between two)
3. Cook for 5 minutes or until you no longer see steam coming from the waffle maker.
4. Remove to a wire rack and allow to cool.

Nutrition:

- Calories: 156 kcal
- Cholesterol: 86 mg
- Carbohydrates: 5.7 g
- Protein: 3.9 g

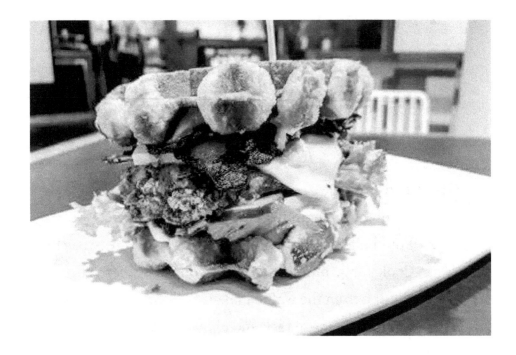

LUNCH CHAFFLE RECIPES

9. Chaffle With Cheese & Bacon

Preparation Time: 10 minutes

Cooking Time: 15 Minutes

Servings: 2

Ingredients:

- 1 egg
- 1/2 cup cheddar cheese, shredded
- 1 tbsp. parmesan cheese
- 3/4 tsp coconut flour
- 1/4 tsp baking powder
- 1/8 tsp Italian Seasoning
- pinch of salt
- 1/4 tsp garlic powder
- For Topping
- 1 bacon sliced, cooked and chopped
- 1/2 cup mozzarella cheese, shredded
- 1/4 tsp parsley, chopped

Directions:

1. Preheat oven to 400 degrees.
2. Switch on your minutes waffle maker and grease with cooking spray.

3. Mix together chaffle ingredients in a mixing bowl until combined.
4. Spoon half of the batter in the center of the waffle maker and close the lid. Cook chaffles for about 3-minutesutes until cooked.
5. Carefully remove chaffles from the maker.
6. Arrange chaffles in a greased baking tray.
7. Top with mozzarella cheese, chopped bacon and parsley.
8. And bake in the oven for 4 -5 minutes Utes.
9. Once the cheese is melted, remove from the oven.
10. Serve and enjoy!

Nutrition:

- Protein: 28% 90 kcal
- Fat: 69% 222 kcal
- Carbohydrates: 3% kcal

10. Grill Beefsteak and Chaffle

Preparation Time: 10 minutes

Cooking Time: 10 Minutes

Servings: 1

Ingredients:

- 1 beefsteak rib eye
- 1 tsp salt
- 1 tsp pepper
- 1 tbsp. lime juice
- 1 tsp garlic

Directions:

1. Prepare your grill for direct heat.
2. Mix together all spices and rub over beefsteak evenly.
3. Place the beef on the grill rack over medium heat.
4. Cover and cook steak for about6 to 8 minutes Utes. Flip and cook for another 5 minutes Utes until cooked through.
5. Serve with keto simple chaffle and enjoy!

Nutrition:

- Protein: 51% 274 kcal
- Fat: 45% 243 kcal
- Carbohydrates: 4% 22 kcal

11. Cauliflower Chaffles And Tomatoes

Preparation Time: 10 minutes

Cooking Time: 15 Minutes

Servings: 2

Ingredients:

- 1/2 cup cauliflower
- 1/4 tsp. garlic powder
- 1/4 tsp. black pepper
- 1/4 tsp. Salt
- 1/2 cup shredded cheddar cheese
- 1 egg
- For Topping
- 1 lettuce leave
- 1 tomato sliced
- 4 oz. cauliflower steamed, mashed
- 1 tsp sesame seeds

Directions:

1. Add all chaffle ingredients into a blender and mix well.
2. Sprinkle 1/8 shredded cheese on the waffle maker and pour cauliflower mixture in a preheated waffle maker and sprinkle the rest of the cheese over it.
3. Cook chaffles for about 4-5 minutes Utes until cooked

4. For serving, lay lettuce leaves over chaffle top with steamed cauliflower and tomato.
5. Drizzle sesame seeds on top.
6. Enjoy!

Nutrition:
- Protein: 25% 49 kcal
- Fat: 65% 128 kcal
- Carbohydrates: 10% 21 kcal

12. Rosemary Pork Chops in Chaffles

Preparation Time: 10 minutes

Cooking Time: 15 Minutes

Servings: 2

Ingredients:

- 4 eggs
- 2 cups grated mozzarella cheese
- Salt and pepper to taste
- Pinch of nutmeg
- 2 tablespoons sour cream
- 6 tablespoons almond flour
- 2 teaspoons baking powder
- Pork chops
- 2 tablespoons olive oil
- 1 pound pork chops
- Salt and pepper to taste
- 1 teaspoon freshly chopped rosemary
- Other
- 2 tablespoons cooking spray to brush the waffle maker
- 2 tablespoons freshly chopped basil for decoration

Directions:

1. Preheat the waffle maker.

2. Add the eggs, mozzarella cheese, salt and pepper, nutmeg, sour cream, almond flour and baking powder to a bowl.

3. Mix until combined.

4. Brush the heated waffle maker with cooking spray and add a few tablespoons of the batter.

5. Close the lid and cook for about 7 minutes depending on your waffle maker.

6. Meanwhile, heat the butter in a nonstick grill pan and season the pork chops with salt and pepper and freshly chopped rosemary.

7. Cook the pork chops for about 4 5 minutes on each side.

8. Serve each chaffle with a pork chop and sprinkle some freshly chopped basil on top.

Nutrition:

- Calories 666 kcal
- Fat 55.2 g
- Carbs 4.8 g
- Sugar 0.4 g
- Protein 37.5 g
- Sodium 235 mg

13. Classic Beef Chaffle

Preparation Time: 10 minutes
Cooking Time: 10 Minutes
Servings: 2
Ingredients:

- Batter
- ½ pound ground beef
- 4 eggs
- 4 ounces cream cheese
- 1 cup grated mozzarella cheese
- Salt and pepper to taste
- 1 clove garlic, minced
- ½ teaspoon freshly chopped rosemary
- Other
- 2 tablespoons butter to brush the waffle maker
- ¼ cup sour cream
- 2 tablespoons freshly chopped parsley for garnish

Directions:

1. Preheat the waffle maker.
2. Add the ground beef, eggs, cream cheese, grated mozzarella cheese, salt and pepper, minced garlic and freshly chopped rosemary to a bowl.
3. Brush the heated waffle maker with butter and add a few tablespoons of the batter.

4. Close the lid and cook for about 8–10 minutes depending on your waffle maker.
5. Serve each chaffle with a tablespoon of sour cream and freshly chopped parsley on top.
6. Serve and enjoy.

Nutrition:

- Calories 368 kcal
- Fat 24 g
- Carbs 2.1 g
- Sugar 0.4 g
- Protein 27.4 g
- Sodium 291 mg

14. Beef and Tomato Chaffle

Preparation Time: 10 minutes
Cooking Time: 15 Minutes
Servings: 2
Ingredients:

- Batter
- 4 eggs
- ¼ cup cream cheese
- 1 cup grated mozzarella cheese
- Salt and pepper to taste
- ¼ cup almond flour
- 1 teaspoon freshly chopped dill
- Beef
- 1 pound beef loin
- Salt and pepper to taste
- 1 tablespoon balsamic vinegar
- 2 tablespoons olive oil
- 1 teaspoon freshly chopped rosemary
- Other
- 2 tablespoons cooking spray to brush the waffle maker
- 4 tomato slices for serving

Directions:

1. Preheat the waffle maker.
2. Add the eggs, cream cheese, grated mozzarella cheese, salt and pepper, almond flour and freshly chopped dill to a bowl.
3. Mix until combined and batter forms.
4. Brush the heated waffle maker with cooking spray and add a few tablespoons of the batter.
5. Close the lid and cook for about 8–10 minutes depending on your waffle maker.
6. Meanwhile, heat the olive oil in a nonstick frying pan and season the beef loin with salt and pepper and freshly chopped rosemary.
7. Cook the beef on each side for about 5 minutes and drizzle with some balsamic vinegar.
8. Serve each chaffle with a slice of tomato and cooked beef loin slices.

Nutrition:

- Calories 4 kcal
- Fat 35.8 g
- Carbs 3.3 g
- Sugar 0.8 g
- Protein 40.3 g
- Sodium 200 mg

15. Classic Ground Pork Chaffle

Preparation Time: 10 minutes

Cooking Time: 15 Minutes

Servings: 2

Ingredients:

- ½ pound ground pork
- 3 eggs
- ½ cup grated mozzarella cheese
- Salt and pepper to taste
- 1 clove garlic, minced
- 1 teaspoon dried oregano
- Other
- 2 tablespoons butter to brush the waffle maker
- 2 tablespoons freshly chopped parsley for garnish

Directions:

1. Preheat the waffle maker.
2. Add the ground pork, eggs, mozzarella cheese, salt and pepper, minced garlic and dried oregano to a bowl.
3. Mix until combined.
4. Brush the heated waffle maker with butter and add a few tablespoons of the batter.
5. Close the lid and cook for about 7–8 minutes depending on your waffle maker.
6. Serve with freshly chopped parsley.

Nutrition:

- Calories 192 kcal
- Fat 11.g
- Carbs 1 g
- Sugar 0.3 g
- Protein 20.2 g
- Sodium 142 mg

16. Spicy Jalapeno Popper Chaffles

Preparation Time: 10 mins

Cooking Time: 10 mins

Servings: 1

Ingredients:

- for the chaffles:
- 1 egg
- 1 oz cream cheese, softened
- 1 cup cheddar cheese, shredded
- For the toppings:
- 2 tbsp bacon bits
- 1/2 tbsp jalapenos

Directions:

1. Turn on the waffle maker. Preheat for up to 5 minutes.
2. Mix the chaffle Ingredients.
3. Pour the batter onto the waffle maker.
4. Cook the batter for 3-4 minutes until it's brown and crispy.
5. Remove the chaffle and repeat steps until all remaining batter have been used up.
6. Sprinkle bacon bits and a few jalapeno slices as toppings.

Nutrition:

- Calories: 231 kcal
- Carbohydrate: 2g
- Fat: 18g
- Protein: 13g

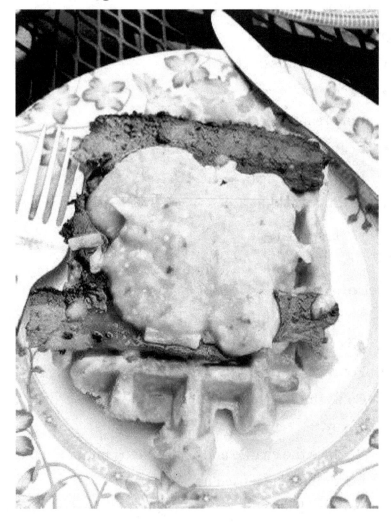

DINNER CHAFFLE RECIPES

17.   Turkey Chaffle Sandwich

Preparation Time: 10 minutes

Cooking Time: 15 Minutes

Servings: 2

Ingredients:

- Batter
- 4 eggs
- ¼ cup cream cheese
- 1 cup grated mozzarella cheese
- Salt and pepper to taste
- 1 teaspoon dried dill
- ½ teaspoon onion powder
- ½ teaspoon garlic powder
- Juicy chicken
- 2 tablespoons butter
- 1 pound chicken breast
- Salt and pepper to taste
- 1 teaspoon dried dill
- 2 tablespoons heavy cream
- Other
- 2 tablespoons butter to brush the waffle maker
- 4 lettuce leaves to garnish the sandwich
- 4 tomato slices to garnish the sandwich

Directions:

1. Preheat the waffle maker.
2. Add the eggs, cream cheese, mozzarella cheese, salt and pepper, dried dill, onion powder and garlic powder to a bowl.
3. Mix everything with a fork just until batter forms.
4. Brush the heated waffle maker with butter and add a few tablespoons of the batter.
5. Close the lid and cook for about 7 minutes depending on your waffle maker.
6. Meanwhile, heat some butter in a nonstick pan.
7. Season the chicken with salt and pepper and sprinkle with dried dill. Pour the heavy cream on top.
8. Cook the chicken slices for about 10 minutes or until golden brown.
9. Cut each chaffle in half.
10. On one half add a lettuce leaf, tomato slice, and chicken slice. Cover with the other chaffle half to make a sandwich.
11. Serve and enjoy.

Nutrition:

- Calories: 350 kcal
- Protein: 51 g
- Carbohydrates: 10 g
- Fats: 10 g

18. BBQ Sauce Pork Chaffle

Preparation Time: 10 minutes

Cooking Time: 15 Minutes

Servings: 2

Ingredients:

- ½ pound ground pork
- 3 eggs
- 1 cup grated mozzarella cheese
- Salt and pepper to taste
- 1 clove garlic, minced
- 1 teaspoon dried rosemary
- 3 tablespoons sugar-free BBQ sauce
- Other
- 2 tablespoons butter to brush the waffle maker
- ½ pound pork rinds for serving
- ¼ cup sugar-free BBQ sauce for serving

Directions:

1. Preheat the waffle maker.
2. Add the ground pork, eggs, mozzarella, salt and pepper, minced garlic, dried rosemary, and BBQ sauce to a bowl.
3. Mix until combined.
4. Brush the heated waffle maker with butter and add a few tablespoons of the batter.

5. Close the lid and cook for about 7–8 minutes depending on your waffle maker.

6. Serve each chaffle with some pork rinds and a tablespoon of BBQ sauce.

Nutrition:

- Calories: 529 kcal
- Protein: 34 g
- Carbohydrates: 68 g
- Fats: 13 g

19. Chicken Taco Chaffle

Preparation Time: 10 minutes
Cooking Time: 15 Minutes
Servings: 2
Ingredients:

- Batter
- 4 eggs
- 2 cups grated provolone cheese
- 6 tablespoons almond flour
- 2½ teaspoons baking powder
- Salt and pepper to taste
- Chicken topping
- 2 tablespoons olive oil
- ½ pound ground chicken
- Salt and pepper to taste
- 1 garlic clove, minced
- 2 teaspoons dried oregano
- Other
- 2 tablespoons butter to brush the waffle maker
- 2 tablespoons freshly chopped spring onion for garnishing

Directions:

1. Preheat the waffle maker.
2. Add the eggs, grated provolone cheese, almond flour, baking powder and salt and pepper to a bowl.
3. Mix until just combined.
4. Brush the heated waffle maker with cooking spray and add a few tablespoons of the batter.
5. Close the lid and cook for about 7–9 minutes depending on your waffle maker.
6. Meanwhile, heat the olive oil in a nonstick pan over medium heat and start cooking the ground chicken.
7. Season with salt and pepper and stir in the minced garlic and dried oregano. Cook for 10 minutes.
8. Add some of the cooked ground chicken to each chaffle and serve with freshly chopped spring onion.

Nutrition:

- Calories: 350 kcal
- Protein: 51 g
- Carbohydrates: 10 g
- Fats: 10 g

20. Italian Chicken and Basil Chaffles

Preparation Time: 10 minutes

Cooking Time: 7–9 Minutes

Servings: 2

Ingredients:

- Batter
- ½ pound ground chicken
- 4 eggs
- 3 tablespoons tomato sauce
- Salt and pepper to taste
- 1 cup grated mozzarella cheese
- 1 teaspoon dried oregano
- 3 tablespoons freshly chopped basil leaves
- ½ teaspoon dried garlic
- Other
- 2 tablespoons butter to brush the waffle maker
- ¼ cup tomato sauce for serving
- 1 tablespoon freshly chopped basil for serving

Directions:

1. Preheat the waffle maker.
2. Add the ground chicken, eggs and tomato sauce to a bowl and season with salt and pepper.

3. Add the mozzarella cheese and season with dried oregano, freshly chopped basil and dried garlic.
4. Mix until fully combined and batter forms.
5. Brush the heated waffle maker with butter and add a few tablespoons of the chaffle batter.
6. Close the lid and cook for about 7–9 minutes depending on your waffle maker.
7. Repeat with the rest of the batter.
8. Serve with tomato sauce and freshly chopped basil on top.

Nutrition:

- Calories: 350 kcal
- Protein: 51 g
- Carbohydrates: 10 g
- Fats: 10 g

21.   Beef Meatballs on Chaffle

Preparation Time: 10 minutes

Cooking Time: 20 Minutes

Servings: 2

Ingredients:

- Batter
- 4 eggs
- 2½ cups grated gouda cheese
- ¼ cup heavy cream
- Salt and pepper to taste
- 1 spring onion, finely chopped
- Beef meatballs
- 1 pound ground beef
- Salt and pepper to taste
- 2 teaspoons Dijon mustard
- 1 spring onion, finely chopped
- 5 tablespoons almond flour
- 2 tablespoons butter
- Other
- 2 tablespoons cooking spray to brush the waffle maker
- 2 tablespoons freshly chopped parsley

Directions:

1. Preheat the waffle maker.
2. Add the eggs, grated gouda cheese, heavy cream, salt and pepper and finely chopped spring onion to a bowl.
3. Mix until combined and batter forms.
4. Brush the heated waffle maker with cooking spray and add a few tablespoons of the batter.
5. Close the lid and cook for about 7 minutes depending on your waffle maker.
6. Meanwhile, mix the ground beef meat, salt and pepper, Dijon mustard, chopped spring onion and almond flour in a large bowl.
7. Form small meatballs with your hands.
8. Heat the butter in a nonstick frying pan and cook the beef meatballs for about 3–4 minutes on each side.
9. Serve each chaffle with a couple of meatballs and some freshly chopped parsley on top.

Nutrition:

- Calories: 350 kcal
- Protein: 51 g
- Carbohydrates: 10 g
- Fats: 10 g

22. Leftover Turkey Chaffle

Preparation Time: 10 minutes

Cooking Time: 7–9 Minutes

Servings: 2

Ingredients:

- Batter
- ½ pound shredded leftover turkey meat
- 4 eggs
- 1 cup grated provolone cheese
- Salt and pepper to taste
- 1 teaspoon dried basil
- ½ teaspoon dried garlic
- 3 tablespoons sour cream
- 2 tablespoons coconut flour
- Other
- 2 tablespoons cooking spray for greasing the chaffle maker
- ¼ cup cream cheese for serving the chaffles

Directions:

1. Preheat the waffle maker.
2. Add the leftover turkey, eggs and provolone cheese to a bowl and season with salt and pepper, dried basil and dried garlic.

3. Add the sour cream and coconut flour and mix until batter forms.
4. Brush the heated waffle maker with cooking spray and add a few tablespoons of the chaffle batter.
5. Close the lid and cook for about 7–9 minutes depending on your waffle maker.
6. Repeat with the rest of the batter.
7. Serve with cream cheese on top of each chaffle.

Nutrition:

- Calories: 250 kcal
- Carbohydrates: 14.5 g
- Fats: 15.9 g
- Protein: 25 g

23. Beef Meatza Chaffle

Preparation Time: 10 minutes
Cooking Time: 15 Minutes
Servings: 2
Ingredients:

- Meatza chaffle batter
- ½ pound ground beef
- 4 eggs
- 2 cups grated cheddar cheese
- Salt and pepper to taste
- 1 teaspoon Italian seasoning
- 2 tablespoons tomato sauce
- Other
- 2 tablespoons cooking spray to brush the waffle maker
- ¼ cup tomato sauce for serving
- 2 tablespoons freshly chopped basil for serving

Directions:

1. Preheat the waffle maker.
2. Add the ground beef, eggs, grated cheddar cheese, salt and pepper, Italian seasoning and tomato sauce to a bowl.
3. Mix until everything is fully combined.
4. Brush the heated waffle maker with cooking spray and add a few tablespoons of the batter.

5. Close the lid and cook for about 7–10 minutes depending on your waffle maker.
6. Serve with tomato sauce and freshly chopped basil on top.

Nutrition:

- Calories: 384 kcal
- Protein: 7 g
- Carbohydrates: 22 g
- Fats: 28 g

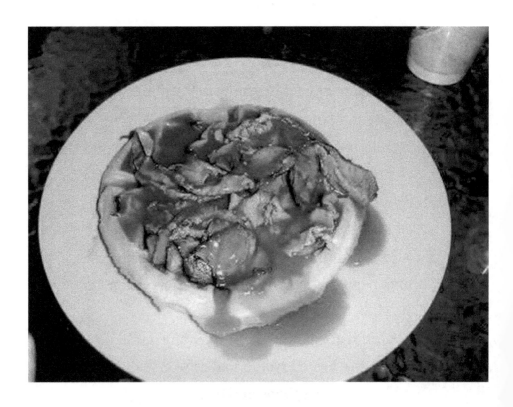

24. Chicken Jalapeno Chaffle

Preparation Time: 10 minutes

Cooking Time: 8–10 Minutes

Servings: 2

Ingredients:

- Batter
- ½ pound ground chicken
- 4 eggs
- 1 cup grated mozzarella cheese
- 2 tablespoons sour cream
- 1 green jalapeno, chopped
- Salt and pepper to taste
- 1 teaspoon dried oregano
- ½ teaspoon dried garlic
- Other
- 2 tablespoons butter to brush the waffle maker
- ¼ cup sour cream to garnish
- 1 green jalapeno, diced, to garnish

Directions:

1. Preheat the waffle maker.
2. Add the ground chicken, eggs, mozzarella cheese, sour cream, chopped jalapeno, salt and pepper, dried oregano and dried garlic to a bowl.

3. Mix everything until batter forms.
4. Brush the heated waffle maker with butter and add a few tablespoons of the batter.
5. Close the lid and cook for about 8–10 minutes depending on your waffle maker.
6. Serve with a tablespoon of sour cream and sliced jalapeno on top.

Nutrition:

- Calories: 502 kcal
- Protein: 6 g
- Carbohydrates: 65 g
- Fats: 24 g

SNACK CHAFFLE RECIPES

25. Chaffle Beacon Sandwich

Preparation Time: 5 minutes

Cooking Time: 25 minutes

Servings: 2

Ingredients:

- 1/2 cup of mozzarella cheese
- 2 Strips of bacon (either pork or beef)
- 2 Tbsp coconut flour
- 2 Tbsp coconut oil
- 2 slice of cheddar cheese
- 1 egg

Directions:

1. In a bowl, add egg, mozzarella, and flour. Mix the ingredients.
2. Preheat the waffle machine, sprinkle cheese and allow to melt. Pour the mixture and cook for 3-4minutes.
3. In a pan, heat coconut oil, add your bacon and fry for 2-3minutes per side, or until it is crispy.
4. Arrange the bacon and cheese on your chaffle, enjoy.

Nutrition:

- Calorie: 295kcal
- Carbs: 2.6g
- Fats: 24.2g
- Protein: 30 g

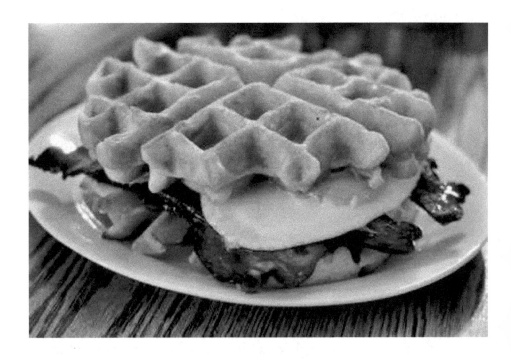

26. Sausage Ball Chaffle

This meal can be eaten as a main meal or side dish. It is tasty, delicious, and also effortless to prepare.

Preparation Time: 5 minutes

Cooking Time: 20 minutes

Servings: 1

Ingredients:

- 1 egg
- 1/2 lb. Of Italian sausage
- 1/4 cup of parmesan cheese
- 2 Tbsp of flour
- 1 cup of cheddar cheese (grated)
- 1 tsp of baking powder

Directions:

1. In a bowl, combine the egg, flour, baking powder, and Italian sausage. Mix well.
2. Preheat the waffle-maker, sprinkle parmesan cheese and allow to cook for about 30 seconds.
3. Pour in the sausage mixture, close, and allow to cook for 3-4minutes or until it turns golden brown.
4. Serve hot.

Nutrition:

- Calorie: 245kcal
- Carbs: 1.1 g
- Fats: 13.4g
- Protein: 19.1g

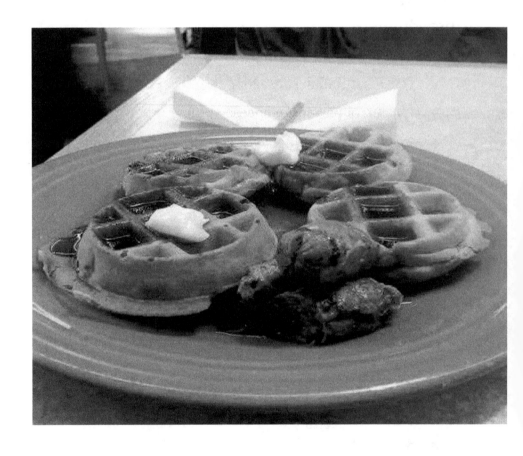

27. Parmesan Chicken Filled Chaffle

Preparation Time: 5 minutes

Cooking Time: 15 minutes

Servings: 2

Ingredients:

- 2 slices of parmesan cheese
- 1/2 cup of chicken breast (shredded)
- 1/4 cup of parmesan cheese
- 1 Tbsp of Pizza sauce
- 1 Egg
- 1/4 cup of mozzarella cheese
- 1 tsp of thick cream cheese
- 1/4 tsp of garlic powder
- 1/4 tsp of Italian seasoning

Directions:

1. In a bowl, combine the shredded chicken, garlic powder, Italian seasoning, mozzarella, parmesan, cream cheese, egg, and mix until smooth.
2. Preheat your waffle-maker, sprinkle some cheese on top. Leave for seconds, pour the chicken mixture, and sprinkle some cheese. Close the waffle-maker.
3. Cook the chaffle for 3-5 minutes or until it turns golden brown. Remove and spread pizza sauce on top, add the

parmesan cheese slice (make sure the chaffle is until hot when adding the cheese to allow it to melt).

4. Serve hot.

Nutrition:

- Calorie: 225kcal
- Carbs: 2.1g
- Fats: 8.3g
- Protein: 9.3g

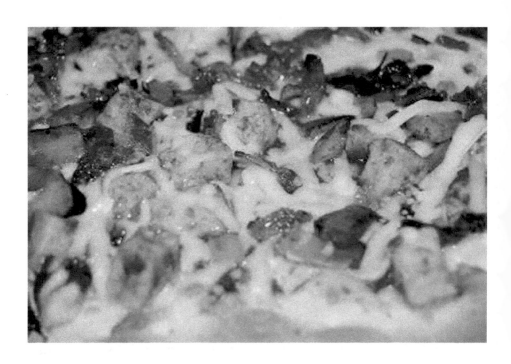

28. Zucchini Chaffle

Preparation Time: 5 minutes

Cooking Time: 25 minutes

Servings: 2

Ingredients:

- 1 zucchini (grated)
- 2 eggs
- 1/2 cup of Cheddar cheese (shredded)
- 1 clove of garlic (mashed)
- 2 pinches of salt
- 1/4 cup of diced onion

Directions:

1. In a bowl, add the egg, grated zucchini, onions, and garlic. Mix well.
2. Preheat the waffle-maker, add cheese and allow it to melt. Add the mixture, sprinkle more cheese, and allow to cook for 3-5 minutes or until it turns golden brown.
3. Serve hot.

Nutrition:

- Calorie: 170 kcal
- Carbs: 4g
- Fats: 10g
- Protein: 13g

29. Keto Chocolate Chaffle

Preparation Time: 5 minutes

Cooking Time: 15 minutes

Servings: 2

Ingredients:

- 1 tsp vanilla extract
- 1 egg
- 1 tsp of cocoa powder
- 3/4 oz. Cream cheese
- 1-1/2 Tbsp coconut flour

Directions:

1. In a bowl, add all the ingredients and mix thoroughly.
2. Preheat the waffle-maker, pour the mixture and allow to cook for 3-4minutes or until it turns golden brown.
3. Serve hot.

Nutrition:

- Calorie: 230kcal
- Carbs: 4g
- Fats: 10g
- Protein: 13g

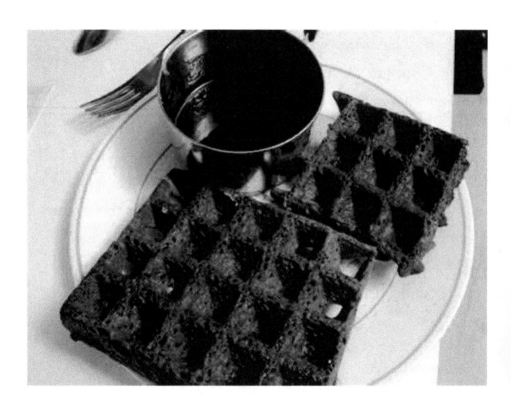

30. Jalapeno Chicken Popper Chaffles

Preparation Time: 5 minutes

Cooking Time: 15 minutes

Servings: 2

Ingredients:

- 1/2 cup of chicken (shredded)
- 1/4 cup of mozzarella cheese
- 1/4 tsp of garlic powder
- 1/4 cup of parmesan cheese
- 1/4 tsp of onion powder
- 1 fresh jalapeno (diced)
- 1 egg
- 1 tsp of cream cheese

Directions:

1. Preheat the waffle-maker.
2. In a bowl, add all the ingredients and mix thoroughly.
3. Sprinkle cheese on the waffle-maker and heat for 20 seconds. Pour the mixture on top and allow it to cook for 3-4 minutes.
4. Serve with any sauce or toppings of choice

Nutrition:

- Calorie: 231.4kcal
- Carbs: 4.5g
- Fats: 10.6g
- Protein: 19.2g

31. Cauliflower Chaffle

Preparation Time: 5 minutes

Cooking Time: 25 minutes

Servings: 2

Ingredients:

- 1/4 cup of diced chicken thigh (into cubes)
- 1 Clove of garlic (mashed)
- 1 cup of cauliflower (shredded and pre-cooked)
- 1/2 cup of mozzarella cheese (shredded)
- 1/2 tsp of black pepper (grounded)
- 1/2 cup of parmesan cheese
- 1/2 tsp of soy sauce
- 1/2 stalk of green onion
- 1 egg

Directions:

1. In a blender, add the cauliflower, egg, mozzarella cheese, garlic, and pepper. Blend the ingredients and pour the mixture into a bowl.
2. Preheat the waffle-maker, sprinkle parmesan cheese.
3. Add soy sauce and diced chicken to the cauliflower mixture, then mix well.
4. Pour the mixture over the melted cheese, sprinkle parmesan cheese, and cook for 4-5 minutes.
5. Serve hot.

Nutrition:

- Calorie: 256kcal
- Carbs: 5.8g
- Fats: 15.6g
- Protein: 21g

32. Sloppy Joe Chaffle

Preparation Time: 5 minutes

Cooking Time: 20 minutes

Servings: 2

Ingredients:

- 1/4-pound ground beef
- 1 egg
- 2 Tbsp of tomato paste
- 1/2 cup of cheddar cheese
- 1/4 cup onions (diced)
- 1 tsp of garlic paste
- 1/2 tsp of pepper
- 1/2 cup of broth
- 1/2 tsp of salt
- 2 tsp soy sauce
- 1/2 tsp paprika
- 2 tsp coconut oil
- 1/2 tsp of mustard sauce
- 1/2 tsp cocoa powder

Directions:

1. Place a pot over medium heat, add coconut oil and garlic paste. Sauté for 1 minute, then add the grounded beef, salt, and pepper. Allow it to cook for 2-3 minutes.

2. Add the tomato paste, paprika, soy sauce, cocoa powder, mustard sauce, and the broth. Cook for 1minute then simmer the mixture.

3. Preheat the waffle-maker. In a bowl, whisk egg and cheese.

4. Sprinkle cheese on the waffle-maker, pour the mixture and allow to cook for 3-4 minutes.

5. Arrange the beef mixture on your chaffle and serve.

Nutrition:

- Calorie: 198kcal
- Carbs: 3 1g
- Fats: 8.4g
- Protein: 6g

OTHER KETO CHAFFLE RECIPES

33. Simple Chaffles With Cream Dip

Preparation Time: 9 minutes

Cooking Time: 10 Minutes

Servings: 2

Ingredients:

- Chaffles
- 1 organic egg, beaten
- 2 tablespoons almond flour
- ½ teaspoon organic baking powder
- ½ cup mozzarella cheese, shredded
- Dip
- ¼ cup heavy whipping cream
- 1-2 drops liquid stevia

Directions:

1. Preheat a mini waffle iron and then grease it.
2. For chaffles: In a medium bowl, put all ingredients and with a fork, mix until well combined. Place half of the mixture into preheated waffle iron and cook for about 3–5 minutes.

3. Repeat with the remaining mixture.
4. Meanwhile, for dip: in a bowl, mix together the cream and stevia.
5. Serve warm chaffles alongside the cream dip.

Nutrition:

- Calories 149 kcal
- Net Carbs 1.9 g
- Total Fat 12.8 g
- Saturated Fat 5.1 g
- Cholesterol 10mg
- Sodium 80 mg
- Total Carbs 2.7 g
- Fiber 0.8 g
- Sugar 0.4 g
- Protein 5.1 g

34. Raspberry Chaffle

Preparation Time: 5 minutes

Cooking Time: 8 Minutes

Servings: 2

Ingredients:

- 1 large egg (beaten)
- 1 tsp cinnamon
- 2 tbsp cream cheese
- ½ tsp vanilla extract
- 2 tbsp heavy cream
- 2 tbsp almond flour
- ¼ tsp baking powder
- 1/3 cup raspberries
- 2 tsp swerve sweetener or to taste
- 1/8 tsp salt

Directions:

1. Plug the waffle maker to preheat it and spray it with a non-stick spray.
2. In a medium mixing bowl, combine the cinnamon, almond flour, baking powder, 1 tsp swerve and salt.
3. In another mixing bowl, combine the cream cheese, egg and vanilla extract.

4. Pour the cream cheese mixture into the cheese mixture and mix until well combine and you have formed a smooth batter.
5. Fold in half of the raspberries.
6. Fill the waffle maker with an appropriate amount of the batter. Spread out the batter to cover all the holes on the waffle maker.
7. Close the waffle maker and cook for about 3-4 minutes or according to waffle maker's settings.
8. After the cooking cycle, use a plastic or silicone utensil to remove the chaffle from the waffle maker.
9. Repeat 6 to 7 until you have cooked all the batter into chaffles.
10. In a mixing bowl, combine the remaining swerve and heavy cream. Whisk until you form soft peak.
11. Spread the cream cheese mixture over the chaffles and top with the remaining raspberries.
12. Serve and enjoy.

Nutrition:

- Fat 30.4g 39%
- Carbohydrate 16.4g 6%
- Sugars 3.1g
- Protein 12g

35. Choco Peanut Butter Chaffle

Preparation Time: 9 minutes

Cooking Time: 10 Minutes

Servings: 2

Ingredients:
- Filling:
- 3 tbsp all-natural peanut butter
- 2 tsp swerve sweetener
- 1 tsp vanilla extract
- 2 tbsp heavy cream
- Chaffle:
- ¼ tsp baking powder
- 1 tbsp unsweetened cocoa powder
- 4 tsp almond flour
- ½ tsp vanilla extract
- 1 tbsp granulated swerve sweetener
- 1 large egg (beaten)
- 1 tbsp heavy cream

Directions:
1. For the chaffle:
2. Plug the waffle maker and preheat it. Spray it with a non-stick spray.
3. In a large mixing bowl, combine the almond flour, cocoa powder, baking powder and swerve.

4. Add the egg, vanilla extract and heavy cream. Mix until the ingredients are well combined and you form a smooth batter.
5. Pour some of the batter into the preheated waffle maker. Spread out the batter to the edges of the waffle maker to cover all the holes on the waffle iron.
6. Close the lid of the waffle iron and bake for about 5 minutes or according to waffle maker's settings.
7. After the baking cycle, use a plastic or silicone utensil to remove the chaffle from the waffle maker.
8. Repeat step 4 to 6 until you have cooked all the batter into chaffles.
9. Transfer the chaffles to a wire rack and let the chaffles cool completely.
10. For the filling:
11. Combine the vanilla, swerve, heavy cream and peanut butter in a bowl. Mix until the ingredients are well combined.
12. Spread the peanut butter frosting over the chaffles and serve.
13. Enjoy.

Nutrition:

- Fat 43.2g 55%
- Carbohydrate 32g12%
- Sugars 9g
- Protein 19g

36. <u>Avocado Chaffles</u>

Preparation Time: 9 minutes

Cooking Time: 5 Minutes

Servings: 2

Ingredients:

- 1 large egg
- 1/2 cup finely shredded mozzarella
- 1/8 cup avocado mash
- 1 tbsp. coconut cream
- TOPPING
- 2 oz. smoked salmon
- 1 Avocado thinly sliced

Directions:

1. Switch on your square waffle maker and grease with cooking spray.
2. Beat egg in a mixing bowl with a fork.
3. Add the cheese, avocado mash and coconut cream to the egg and mix well.
4. Pour chaffle mixture in the preheated waffle maker and cook for about 2-3 minutes Utes.
5. Once chaffles are cooked, carefully remove from the maker.
6. Serve with an avocado slice and smoked salmon.
7. Drizzle ground pepper on top.

8. Enjoy!

Nutrition:

- Protein: 23% kcal
- Fat: 67% 266 kcal
- Carbohydrates: 11% 42 kcal

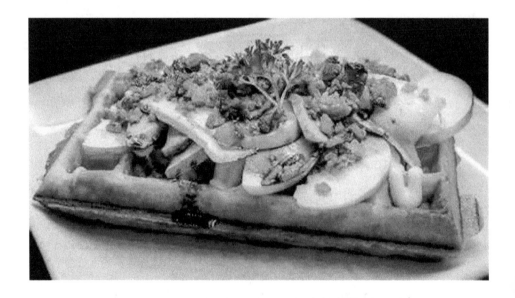

37. Almond Butter Chaffle

Preparation Time: 8 minutes

Cooking Time: 20 Minutes

Servings: 2

Ingredients:

- 2 eggs (beaten)
- 3 tsp granulated swerve sweetener
- 4 tbsp almond flour
- ½ tsp vanilla extract
- ½ cup grated mozzarella cheese
- ½ cup parmesan cheese
- 1/8 tsp allspice
- Almond Butter Filling:
- ½ tsp vanilla extract
- 4 tbsp almond butter
- 2 tbsp butter (melted)
- 2 tbsp swerve sweetener
- 1/8 tsp nutmeg

Directions:

1. Plug the waffle maker to preheat it and spray it with a non-stick cooking spray.
2. In a mixing bowl, combine the mozzarella, allspice, almond flour, and swerve sweetener. Add the egg and

vanilla extract and mix until the ingredients are well combined.

3. Sprinkle some parmesan cheese over the waffle maker.
4. Pour an appropriate amount of the batter into the waffle and spread out the batter to cover all the holes on the waffle maker.
5. Sprinkle some parmesan over the batter.
6. Close the waffle maker and cook for about 5 minutes or according to your waffle maker's settings.
7. After the cooking cycle, use a plastic or silicone utensil to remove the chaffle from the waffle maker. Transfer the chaffle to a wire rack to cool.
8. Repeat step 3 to 7 until you have cooked all the batter into chaffles.
9. For the filling, combine butter, almond butter, swerve, vanilla and nutmeg. Mix until the mixture is smooth and fluffy.
10. Spread the cream over the surface of one chaffle and cover the with another chaffle. Repeat until you have filled all the chaffles.
11. Serve and enjoy.

Nutrition:
- Fat 54.8g 70%
- Carbohydrate 18.4g7%
- Sugars 3.2g
- Protein 29.7g

38. Simple Chaffles Without Maker

Preparation Time: 8 minutes

Cooking Time: 5minutes

Servings: 2

Ingredients:

- 1 tbsp. chia seeds
- 1 egg
- 1/2 cup cheddar cheese
- pinch of salt
- 1 tbsp. avocado oil

Directions:

1. Heat your nonstick pan over medium heat
2. In a small bowl, mix together chia seeds, salt, egg, and cheese together
3. Grease pan with avocado oil.
4. Once the pan is hot, pour 2 tbsps. chaffle batter and cook for about 1-2 minutes Utes.
5. Flip and cook for another 1-2 minutes Utes.
6. Once chaffle is brown remove from pan.
7. Serve with berries on top and enjoy.

Nutrition:

- Protein: 19% 44 kcal
- Fat: % 181 kcal
- Carbohydrates: 1% 2 kcal

39. Heart Shape Chaffles

Preparation Time: 9 minutes

Cooking Time: 5 Minutes

Servings: 2

Ingredients:

- 1 egg
- 1 cup mozzarella cheese
- 1 tsp baking powder
- ¼ cup almond flour
- 1 tbsp. coconut oil

Directions:

1. Heat your nonstick pan over medium heat.
2. Mix together all ingredients in a bowl.
3. Grease pan with avocado oil and place a heart shape cookie cutter over the pan.
4. Once the pan is hot, pour the batter equally in 2 cutters.
5. Cook for another 1-2 minutes Utes.
6. Once chaffle is set, remove the cutter, flip and cook for another 1-2 minutes Utes.
7. Once chaffles are brown, remove from the pan.
8. Serve hot and enjoy!

Nutrition:

- Protein: 24% 43 kcal
- Fat: 6 123 kcal
- Carbohydrates: 6% 11 kcal

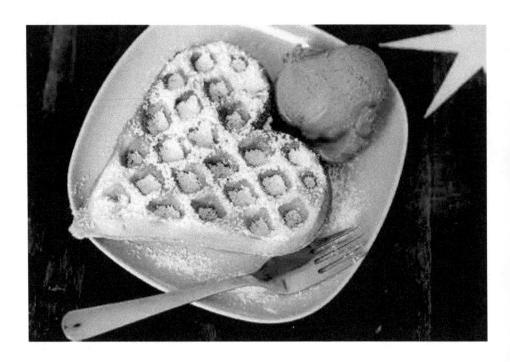

40. Bacon Chaffles With Herb Dip

Preparation Time: 9 minutes

Cooking Time: 10 Minutes

Servings: 2

Ingredients:

- Chaffles
- 1 organic egg, beaten
- ½ cup Swiss/Gruyere cheese blend, shredded
- 2 tablespoons cooked bacon pieces
- 1 tablespoon jalapeño pepper, chopped
- Dip
- ¼ cup heavy cream
- ¼ teaspoon fresh dill, minced
- Pinch of ground black pepper

Directions:

1. Preheat a mini waffle iron and then grease it.
2. For chaffles: In a medium bowl, put all ingredients and mix well.
3. Place half of the mixture into preheated waffle iron and cook for about 5 minutes.
4. Repeat with the remaining mixture.
5. Meanwhile, for dip: in a bowl, mix together the cream and stevia.
6. Serve warm chaffles alongside the dip.

Nutrition:

- Calories 210 kcal
- Net Carbs 2.2 g
- Total Fat 13 g
- Saturated Fat 9.7 g
- Cholesterol 132 mg
- Sodium 164 mg
- Total Carbs 2.3 g
- Fiber 0.1 g
- Sugar 0.7 g
- Protein 11.9 g

CONCLUSION

Chaffles is the amazing new invention you've been waiting for. It's a revolutionary, patent-pending, and 100% vegan protein bar with a thousand uses.

What are chaffles? Chaffles is a delicious new product that can be used to replace the high fat and high sugar snacks in your diet like cheese chips or chocolate bars. It's also gluten-free, vegan, non-GMO, low in sodium and preservative free! The best part is that chaffles taste just as good as candy! You'll never want anything else again after trying this life changing snack.

The combination of protein and savory chaffle taste will keep you wanting to eat more every time. Chaffles are also a great substitute for those times that you feel like having something sweet, but want something healthy with a lot of flavor.

Chaffles come in an assortment of flavors like Pecan Pie or Cherry Pie and can be served with a drizzle of your favorite nut butter or cinnamon sugar for an awesome snack. Or you can create your own combinations by mixing them up the way that makes your mouth water.

Chaffles are great for both kids and adults. They're the perfect snack to bring on a hike for an afternoon treat or to eat on a road trip or flights. Even better, they create a new way for parents to get their kids to eat protein without them even knowing what they're eating. Now if you want your children to enjoy healthy food without complaining, chaffles will be your best friend.

No matter what you eat chaffles with, it will never disappoint! Have it with chicken noodle soup or mashed potatoes for dinner or have it with salad at lunch.

Chaffle is a perfect combination for keto dieters. Besides, keto diet is always low in carbs and high in fat so chaffle is an amazing option for it.

Chaffles are very versatile and can be used as a spread for your favorite bagel or toast, or even on top of a pizza before baking it. You can also use chaffles as an ingredient for your own meals like pancakes, pies, donuts, breads and so much more!

Chaffle comes in two different flavors: savory and sweet. The savory flavor is more of a BBQ flavor while the sweet flavor is more cookie dough style. The savory chaffles are perfect for replacing things like bread and crackers, while sweet chaffles can be used as a dessert or drink! You can also add chaffle to your favorite dessert recipes for an amazing taste.

Chaffles are the most unique tasting protein bar around that is also good for you. You won't believe how good they taste until you try them for yourself. This incredible product is sure to revolutionize your snacking experience and change the way you think about eating healthy forever.

Always remember when making your own chaffle recipes, you can choose from almost any combination of things like fruits, cereals, nuts and seeds. You can even use different types of chocolate in some recipes. Anything goes with chaffle!

What's even more exciting is that chaffles come in many sizes to fit anyone's taste and diet.

It's time to ditch your unhealthy snacks for life changing chaffles!

CPSIA information can be obtained
at www.ICGtesting.com
Printed in the USA
BVHW011158170521
607543BV00007B/1057